VOLTAGE HEALTH

EXPLORING THE LINK BETWEEN CHARGERS AND WELLNESS

Sam Swinton

DISCLAIMER

The information provided in this book is for educational and informational purposes only. It is not intended to substitute for professional medical advice, diagnosis, or treatment. Readers are encouraged to consult with their healthcare provider regarding any health concerns or questions related to phone chargers or their impact on human health. The author and publisher disclaim any liability arising directly or indirectly from the use of the information contained in this book.

TABLE OF CONTENT

INTRODUCTION

Hey there, fellow tech enthusiasts and health aficionados! Get ready to dive into the electrifying world of "Voltage Health: Exploring the Link Between Chargers and Wellness" authored by yours truly, Sam Swinton!

In this book, we're not just talking about your everyday chargers - we're uncovering the shockingly intriguing connection between these devices and our well-being. From the buzzing currents to the ins and outs of charging tech, we'll unravel the mysteries that lie within your power cords.

Ever wondered if your trusty charger could impact your health? Brace yourself for an electrifying journey where we debunk myths, shed light on facts, and spark curiosity about the relationship between chargers and our overall wellness.

So, fellow voltage voyagers, fasten your seatbelts (or maybe your charging cables?) as we embark on an adventure that blends technology, health, and a jolt of excitement. Get ready to charge up your knowledge and power through these electrifying pages!

Let's explore, learn, and, most importantly, stay charged up for a healthier tomorrow!

Spark on!

Sam Swinton

CHAPTER 1: WIRED WORLD: UNDERSTANDING CHARGERS AND TECHNOLOGY

THE EVOLUTION OF CHARGING DEVICES

The modern world thrives on an intricate web of technological marvels, and among them, the evolution of charging devices stands as a testament to human innovation. From the rudimentary roots of basic power supply mechanisms to the sleek, high-speed chargers of today, the journey of charging devices has been a transformative one, revolutionizing the way we power our indispensable gadgets.

In the early days of technological advancement, charging devices were elementary, designed primarily to supply power to simple electronics. The birth of electrical power systems in the late 19th century paved the way for the creation of the first charging mechanisms. These early chargers consisted of direct current (DC) power supplies, often requiring manual connections and possessing limited compatibility.

The mid-20th century witnessed a pivotal shift in charging technology with the advent of alternating current (AC) power sources and the standardization of voltages.

This development not only enhanced the efficiency of charging but also broadened the range of devices that could be powered. As electronics evolved, so did the chargers, becoming more adaptable and standardized, thus setting the stage for the modern charging landscape.

The emergence of portable electronics in the latter part of the 20th century catalyzed a significant evolution in charging devices. The proliferation of devices such as mobile phones, laptops, and portable music players demanded versatile charging solutions. Consequently, manufacturers began developing smaller, more efficient chargers capable of handling various voltages and currents, facilitating the growth of a more interconnected world.

With the dawn of the 21st century, the rapid pace of technological innovation ushered in a new era of charging devices. The demand for faster charging, wireless capabilities, and eco-friendliness became paramount.

As a result, rapid charging technologies such as Quick Charge, Power Delivery, and wireless charging standards like Qi emerged, offering users unprecedented convenience and speed.

Moreover, the call for sustainable practices birthed eco-friendly charging solutions, emphasizing energy efficiency and reduced environmental impact. Solar-powered chargers, energy harvesting technologies, and recyclable materials in charger production became focal points, aligning with the global shift toward sustainability.

Today, charging devices have transcended mere power sources; they've become sophisticated systems employing cutting-edge technology. Smart chargers equipped with advanced circuitry and adaptive features have revolutionized the charging experience, ensuring faster, safer, and more efficient power delivery.

Looking ahead, the evolution of charging devices seems boundless. The integration of artificial intelligence, advancements in material science, and the pursuit of even faster and more convenient charging methods are on the horizon.

Innovations like biodegradable materials, self-regulating chargers, and ubiquitous wireless charging hold promise for a future where charging devices seamlessly integrate into our lives while prioritizing sustainability and efficiency.

The evolution of charging devices from humble beginnings to the sophisticated systems of today mirrors humanity's relentless quest for progress. These devices have not only powered our gadgets but also connected us in ways previously unimaginable. As we stride into the future, charging devices will continue to evolve, empowering our ever-connected world while striving for a harmonious balance between innovation, convenience, and sustainability.

HOW CHARGERS WORK: FROM VOLTAGE TO POWER

In our daily lives, chargers are indispensable tools that power our devices, keeping them functional and at our fingertips. Yet, behind their seemingly simple task lies a fascinating process that converts electrical energy into a usable form for our gadgets. Understanding how chargers work, from voltage to power, unveils the intricate mechanisms that make our devices come to life.

At its core, a charger's primary objective is to deliver electrical energy to rechargeable devices like smartphones, laptops, or tablets. The process begins with the main power source, typically a wall outlet or USB port, which supplies alternating current (AC) electricity. However, most electronic devices require direct current (DC) power for operation and charging. This is where the charger steps in as a vital intermediary.

The charger's first task is to convert the incoming AC electricity into DC electricity.

This transformation occurs through a component called a rectifier, which contains diodes that ensure the current flows in only one direction, converting the AC power into a steady DC output.

Once the electricity is converted into DC, the charger further regulates this power to match the specific voltage and current requirements of the device being charged. Different devices often require different voltage and current levels for optimal charging without damaging the battery.

To adjust the voltage, chargers utilize a transformer or voltage regulator, modifying the electrical potential to match the device's requirements. Simultaneously, the charger's circuitry controls the current flow, ensuring a safe and steady supply of power to the device without overloading it.

Modern chargers also incorporate smart technology or IC (integrated circuits) that communicate with the device being charged. This communication allows the charger to negotiate the ideal charging rate and adapt its output accordingly, optimizing the charging process for efficiency and safety.

Furthermore, certain chargers come equipped with additional features like fast-charging capabilities. These chargers use more sophisticated circuitry, capable of delivering higher currents or voltages to charge devices at a much faster rate without causing damage to the battery.

Wireless chargers, a more recent innovation, operate on the principle of electromagnetic induction. They generate an electromagnetic field that transfers energy to a receiver coil within the device, eliminating the need for physical connectors and enabling convenient, cable-free charging.

In essence, chargers function as intricate translators and regulators of electrical energy, transforming incoming AC power into a suitable DC form while adjusting voltage and current to match the device's needs. This process ensures that our devices receive the precise amount of power required for efficient and safe charging.

Understanding how chargers work, from voltage conversion to power regulation, unveils the complexity behind these seemingly simple devices.

It underscores the importance of efficient and safe charging practices, ensuring that our devices stay powered up while safeguarding their longevity and performance.

TYPES OF CHARGING TECHNOLOGIES

The world of charging technologies has witnessed a remarkable evolution, offering diverse methods to power our devices efficiently and conveniently. From traditional wired connections to innovative wireless solutions, understanding the various types of charging technologies sheds light on the breadth of options available to meet our diverse charging needs.

USB Charging: Universal Serial Bus (USB) charging has become a ubiquitous method for powering numerous devices. USB ports are commonly found on computers, power adapters, and even in vehicles. USB charging standards have evolved over time, with USB Type-A, Type-B, Type-C, and Micro USB being prevalent connectors. The USB Power Delivery (USB-PD) standard enables faster charging by delivering higher power levels through compatible cables and chargers.

Quick Charge: Developed by Qualcomm, Quick Charge technology enhances charging speeds for compatible devices, allowing them to charge significantly faster than conventional methods.

By dynamically adjusting voltage levels, Quick Charge reduces charging times, making it a popular choice for many smartphones and other devices.

Power Delivery (PD): USB Power Delivery is an advanced protocol that allows for higher power transfer and faster charging through USB-C connections. PD supports a wide range of power levels, making it versatile for various devices like laptops, tablets, and smartphones. It enables bidirectional power flow, facilitating not only device charging but also power transfer between devices.

Wireless Charging: Wireless charging technology eliminates the need for physical connectors by transferring power wirelessly through electromagnetic induction or resonance. Qi wireless charging is the most widely adopted standard, enabling devices to charge simply by placing them on a compatible charging pad or surface. This method offers convenience and reduces wear and tear on charging ports.

Fast Wireless Charging: Similar to fast-wired charging, fast wireless charging protocols like Qi fast charging and proprietary technologies from companies like Samsung and Apple deliver higher power levels to compatible devices. This allows for quicker charging compared to standard wireless methods, albeit slightly slower than wired fast-charging solutions.

Solar Charging: Solar-powered chargers utilize photovoltaic cells to convert sunlight into electricity. These chargers are eco-friendly and provide a sustainable charging solution, particularly useful for outdoor activities or situations where access to traditional power sources is limited.

Inductive Charging: This method employs electromagnetic fields to transfer power wirelessly between coils in the charger and the device. It's commonly used in electric toothbrushes, wearable devices, and certain smartphones, offering a convenient way to charge devices without physical contact.

Adaptive Charging: Some chargers come equipped with adaptive charging capabilities, utilizing smart algorithms and sensors to optimize the charging process based on the device's battery health, temperature, and usage patterns. This helps prolong battery life by delivering the right amount of power at the right time.

The array of charging technologies available today reflects ongoing efforts to enhance efficiency, convenience, and sustainability in powering our devices. As technology continues to evolve, these charging methods will likely further improve, offering even faster, safer, and more eco-friendly ways to keep our gadgets powered up and ready for use.

CHAPTER 2: THE HUMAN CIRCUIT: BASICS OF HEALTH AND WELLNESS

INTRODUCTION TO HUMAN HEALTH PARAMETERS

Human health is a complex tapestry woven from various interconnected factors. Understanding and monitoring specific parameters play a pivotal role in assessing an individual's overall well-being. These health parameters, often considered vital indicators, offer valuable insights into an individual's health status, aiding in preventive care, diagnosis, and treatment.

Blood Pressure: One of the fundamental indicators of cardiovascular health, blood pressure measures the force of blood against artery walls during heartbeats (systolic pressure) and between beats (diastolic pressure). High blood pressure (hypertension) can strain the heart and blood vessels, leading to severe health issues like heart disease or stroke.

Heart Rate (Pulse): Heart rate, measured in beats per minute (BPM), indicates the number of times the heart contracts and pumps blood throughout the body. Resting heart rate and changes in heart rate can provide insights into cardiovascular fitness and stress levels.

Body Mass Index (BMI): BMI is a calculation based on an individual's height and weight, providing an estimate of body fat and assessing potential health risks associated with weight. While it's a useful tool, BMI may not accurately reflect body composition for individuals with high muscle mass.

Temperature: Body temperature indicates the body's ability to regulate heat. A normal body temperature range around 98.6°F (37°C). Deviations from this range may indicate infection or other health issues.

Blood Glucose Levels: Glucose levels in the blood reflect the amount of sugar present, essential for providing energy to the body's cells.

Abnormal blood glucose levels, particularly high levels (hyperglycemia) or low levels (hypoglycemia), can indicate diabetes or other metabolic disorders.

Cholesterol Levels: Cholesterol is a fatty substance crucial for various bodily functions. Monitoring levels of high-density lipoprotein (HDL), low-density lipoprotein (LDL), and total cholesterol helps assess cardiovascular health. High LDL levels are linked to increased risk of heart disease.

Respiratory Rate: The number of breaths taken per minute is an indicator of respiratory health. Normal respiratory rates range from 12 to 20 breaths per minute. Changes in respiratory rate can signal respiratory distress or other conditions affecting lung function.

Hydration Status: Adequate hydration is vital for overall health. Monitoring hydration levels through indicators like urine color or volume helps maintain proper bodily functions and prevents dehydration-related complications.

Mental Health Parameters: Mental health is equally important. Assessing factors like mood, sleep patterns, stress levels, and cognitive function contributes to understanding and managing mental well-being.

Physical Fitness Parameters: Parameters like flexibility, strength, endurance, and agility contribute to physical fitness and overall health. Regular exercise and fitness assessments help maintain optimal physical health.

Understanding these human health parameters and regularly monitoring them, either personally or with the assistance of healthcare professionals, forms the cornerstone of proactive health management. By paying attention to these vital indicators, individuals can make informed lifestyle choices, detect potential health issues early, and take necessary steps towards achieving and maintaining a healthy and balanced life.

THE IMPACT OF TECHNOLOGY ON WELL-BEING

In today's interconnected world, technology serves as an integral part of our daily lives, shaping how we communicate, work, learn, and entertain ourselves. While technology has brought about remarkable advancements and conveniences, its pervasive presence also influences our well-being in multifaceted ways, impacting our physical, mental, and social health.

Physical Health:

Sedentary Lifestyle: The prevalence of technology often leads to prolonged periods of sitting, contributing to a sedentary lifestyle. Excessive screen time and decreased physical activity can lead to health issues such as obesity, cardiovascular problems, and musculoskeletal disorders.

Sleep Disruption: The use of electronic devices, particularly before bedtime, can disrupt sleep patterns. The blue light emitted by screens interferes with the body's natural sleep-wake cycle, leading to difficulties falling asleep and affecting the quality of rest.

Tech-related Strain: Continuous use of devices like computers, smartphones, and tablets may cause digital eye strain or computer vision syndrome, characterized by eye discomfort, headaches, and blurred vision.

Mental Health:

Information Overload: The constant influx of information from various digital sources can lead to information overload and cognitive fatigue, impacting attention span, decision-making, and mental clarity.

Social Comparison and Self-esteem: Social media platforms often cultivate an environment of comparison, leading individuals to compare their lives to others' curated online personas. This can negatively impact self-esteem and contribute to feelings of inadequacy or anxiety.

Digital Addiction: Excessive use of technology, especially social media, online gaming, or streaming platforms, can lead to addictive behaviors and dependencies, affecting mental well-being and real-world social interactions.

Social Health:

Digital Disconnect: While technology facilitates connections, excessive reliance on digital communication can lead to a lack of genuine, face-to-face interactions, potentially affecting social skills and relationships.

Cyberbullying and Online Harassment: The anonymity provided by the digital realm can lead to instances of cyberbullying and harassment, adversely affecting mental health and creating social barriers.

Balancing Act:

While acknowledging the potential downsides, technology also offers solutions and benefits that positively impact well-being:

Access to Information and Support: Technology provides access to vast information resources, educational tools, and mental health support services, empowering individuals to seek knowledge and assistance.

Telemedicine and Remote Support: Remote healthcare services and telemedicine platforms allow easier access to medical professionals and mental health support, particularly in remote or underserved areas.

Wellness Apps and Tech Tools: Various apps and devices cater to mental health management, mindfulness, fitness tracking, and sleep improvement, aiding individuals in managing and improving their well-being.

Navigating the impact of technology on well-being requires a balanced approach.

By practicing mindful technology usage, establishing healthy boundaries, and incorporating digital detoxes, individuals can harness the benefits of technology while mitigating its potential adverse effects, paving the way for a healthier and more harmonious relationship with the digital world.

BALANCING TECH USE FOR BETTER HEALTH

In our modern, tech-driven world, finding a harmonious balance between our digital devices and our overall health has become increasingly crucial. While technology offers immense convenience and connectivity, excessive or inappropriate usage can impact our physical, mental, and emotional well-being. Striking a balance between technology use and health involves mindful practices and conscious decision-making to foster a healthier relationship with our digital tools.

Establishing Boundaries:

Set Tech-Free Zones and Times: Designate certain areas or times in your day as tech-free zones or moments. Bedrooms, dining areas during meals, or specific hours before bedtime can be technology-free zones to promote better sleep and enhance real-life interactions.

Limit Screen Time: Set reasonable limits on the amount of time spent on digital devices, especially for leisure activities.

Utilize screen time monitoring tools or apps to track and manage device usage, ensuring a healthier balance between online and offline activities.

Mindful Tech Use:

Practice Digital Mindfulness: Be mindful of your tech usage. Instead of mindlessly scrolling through social media, use technology intentionally for specific purposes, such as learning, connecting with loved ones, or engaging in hobbies.

Take Breaks and Move: Incorporate regular breaks from screens. Use the 20-20-20 rule—every 20 minutes, look at something 20 feet away for 20 seconds—to reduce eye strain. Additionally, stand up, stretch, and move around periodically to combat the effects of a sedentary lifestyle.

Prioritizing Health and Well-being:

Embrace Tech-Free Activities: Engage in tech-free activities that promote well-being, such as reading books, practicing mindfulness or meditation, pursuing hobbies, or spending time in nature.

Focus on Quality Sleep: Create a bedtime routine that involves unplugging from screens at least an hour before sleep. Limiting exposure to blue light allows for better sleep quality, aiding in restorative rest.

Setting Tech-Health Boundaries:

Utilize Health Apps for Monitoring: Leverage health and wellness apps to track fitness goals, monitor sleep patterns, practice meditation, or manage stress. These apps can enhance awareness and encourage healthier habits.

Establish Personal Tech Guidelines: Develop personal guidelines for using technology that align with your health goals. Prioritize mental health by limiting exposure to negative content or engaging in constructive online interactions.

Promoting Digital Detoxes:

Schedule Tech-Free Days: Designate specific days or weekends for digital detoxes. Unplugging from technology during these periods allows for mental rejuvenation and reconnection with real-world experiences.

Engage in Offline Activities: Dedicate time to offline hobbies, social interactions, or activities that foster creativity, relaxation, and personal growth, reducing dependency on screens.

Striking a balance between technology use and health involves conscious choices and intentional actions to create a healthier lifestyle.

By implementing mindful tech practices, setting boundaries, and fostering a healthy tech-life balance, individuals can harness the benefits of technology while prioritizing their overall well-being.

CHAPTER 3: THE CHARGER CONUNDRUM: MYTHS VS. REALITIES

DEBUNKING COMMON MYTHS ABOUT CHARGERS AND HEALTH

In our tech-centric world, chargers play a crucial role in powering our devices, but along with their ubiquity, misconceptions and myths have surfaced regarding their potential impact on human health. Separating fact from fiction is essential to dispel unwarranted concerns and promote a better understanding of the relationship between chargers and our well-being.

Myth 1: Leaving Chargers Plugged In Causes Health Hazards

Reality: One common belief is that leaving chargers plugged in without devices connected may pose health risks due to electromagnetic fields (EMFs) emitted. However, modern chargers are designed to minimize EMF exposure when not actively charging devices. Unplugging chargers when not in use can save energy but is unlikely to significantly impact health.

Myth 2: Overcharging Devices Poses Health Risks

Reality: There's a misconception that overcharging devices, especially overnight, can cause adverse health effects or damage batteries.

Modern devices are equipped with built-in mechanisms that prevent overcharging, rendering this concern largely unfounded. Charging devices overnight is generally safe due to these built-in safety features.

Myth 3: Chargers Emit Harmful Radiation

Reality: Concerns about chargers emitting harmful radiation, particularly when connected to devices, have surfaced. However, the electromagnetic radiation emitted by chargers, including wireless chargers, falls within safe limits regulated by governing bodies. The levels are not considered harmful to human health.

Myth 4: Cheap Chargers Are as Safe as Brand Name Chargers

Reality: Some believe that cheaper, off-brand chargers are as safe and effective as branded ones. In truth, reputable manufacturers adhere to safety standards, ensuring their chargers meet regulatory requirements for electrical safety and quality. Cheap, non-compliant chargers may pose risks like overheating or electrical hazards.

Myth 5: Wireless Chargers Are Harmful Due to Radiation

Reality: Wireless chargers use electromagnetic induction to transfer power, prompting concerns about exposure to radiation. However, studies suggest that the levels of electromagnetic radiation emitted by wireless chargers are within established safety limits and are not known to cause harm to users.

Myth 6: Chargers Emit Dangerous Levels of Heat

Reality: While chargers can generate heat during operation, especially when fast-charging, modern chargers incorporate heat management systems to prevent excessive heat buildup. As long as chargers are used in accordance with manufacturer instructions and are not damaged, they are unlikely to emit dangerous levels of heat.

Myth 7: All Chargers Are Equally Compatible with Devices

Reality: Not all chargers are created equal in terms of compatibility and safety. Using a charger not specifically designed for a device or using counterfeit chargers may result in inefficient charging, damage to the device, or potential safety hazards.

Separating these myths from reality is crucial for informed decision-making and responsible use of chargers. While it's essential to acknowledge potential risks associated with charging devices, adhering to manufacturer guidelines, using certified chargers, and being mindful of safety practices significantly mitigate these concerns.

As technology evolves, focusing on reliable information helps us navigate the ever-changing landscape of chargers and technology while prioritizing our health and safety.

SEPARATING FACT FROM FICTION: CHARGER-RELATED HEALTH CONCERNS

In our tech-driven world, concerns about the potential health impacts of chargers have circulated, often mingling factual information with misconceptions. It's essential to discern fact from fiction regarding charger-related health concerns to make informed decisions about our technology use. By addressing common myths and providing accurate information, we can better understand the real health considerations associated with chargers.

Myth 1: Electromagnetic Fields (EMFs) from Chargers Pose Significant Health Risks

Reality: Electromagnetic fields (EMFs) are emitted by electronic devices, including chargers, but the levels produced by chargers fall well below established safety standards. Scientific research has not conclusively linked exposure to low-level EMFs from chargers to adverse health effects.

Myth 2: Chargers Emit Harmful Radiation

Reality: Chargers do emit electromagnetic radiation, but the radiation levels emitted by chargers, even wireless ones, are within safe limits regulated by health authorities. The radiation emitted by chargers is not classified as ionizing radiation, which is known to cause cell damage.

Myth 3: Charging Devices Near the Body Poses Health Risks

Reality: There are concerns about charging devices near the body, such as keeping a phone in a pocket while charging. While it's advisable to follow manufacturer instructions for safe charging practices, credible studies haven't shown significant health risks associated with using devices while they're charging.

Myth 4: Overcharging Devices Is Harmful to Health

Reality: Overcharging devices, especially with modern electronics, is generally not harmful to health.

Modern devices incorporate mechanisms to prevent overcharging, safeguarding the battery's health. Charging devices overnight, while commonly done, is unlikely to pose significant health risks.

Myth 5: Cheap Chargers Are as Safe as Branded Chargers

Reality: Branded chargers often adhere to safety standards and undergo rigorous testing to meet quality and safety benchmarks. Cheaper, non-certified chargers may lack these safety measures, posing potential risks such as overheating, electrical hazards, or damage to devices.

Myth 6: Chargers Generate Harmful Heat During Operation

Reality: While chargers can generate heat during operation, especially during fast-charging, reputable chargers include built-in heat management systems to prevent overheating. As long as chargers are used according to manufacturer instructions and are undamaged, they are unlikely to emit dangerous levels of heat.

Myth 7: All Chargers Are Interchangeable Across Devices

Reality: Not all chargers are universally compatible with different devices. Using an incompatible or counterfeit charger may lead to inefficient charging, potential damage to devices, or safety hazards. It's advisable to use chargers recommended or provided by the device manufacturer.

By dispelling these myths and clarifying the factual aspects of charger-related health concerns, we can make informed decisions about our technology usage. Adhering to manufacturer guidelines, using certified chargers, and being mindful of safety practices significantly reduce potential risks associated with chargers, ensuring a safer and more informed approach to utilizing technology in our daily lives.

UNDERSTANDING ELECTROMAGNETIC FIELDS (EMFS)

Electromagnetic fields (EMFs) are a fundamental aspect of our natural and technological environments, yet misconceptions and concerns often swirl around them. Understanding EMFs, their sources, and their impact on our surroundings is essential to navigate the complex relationship between these fields and our health.

What Are Electromagnetic Fields (EMFs)?

Electromagnetic fields are invisible areas of energy created by the movement of electrically charged particles. They consist of electric fields (created by voltage) and magnetic fields (created by the flow of electric current). EMFs exist on a spectrum, with frequencies ranging from extremely low frequencies (ELF) to radio frequencies (RF) and higher energy forms like gamma rays and X-rays.

Sources of EMFs:

Natural Sources: EMFs occur naturally in the environment.

The Earth itself generates a magnetic field, and cosmic rays from the sun contribute to natural EMFs.

Man-made Sources: Modern technology, including power lines, electrical wiring, household appliances, wireless devices, and telecommunication towers, also generates EMFs.

Types of EMFs:

Extremely Low Frequency (ELF) EMFs: These are generated by power lines, electrical wiring, and appliances like refrigerators or hairdryers. ELF EMFs have lower frequencies and are often considered non-ionizing, meaning they don't have enough energy to break chemical bonds or cause direct damage to cells.

Radiofrequency (RF) EMFs: RF EMFs come from wireless devices like cell phones, Wi-Fi routers, and Bluetooth devices. They have higher frequencies and are also considered non-ionizing. The concerns around RF EMFs largely revolve around thermal effects due to prolonged exposure.

Health Considerations and Controversies:

The potential health effects of EMFs have been a topic of debate and research for decades. Some studies suggest a possible association between prolonged exposure to certain EMFs, particularly RF EMFs, and health concerns such as:

Increased risk of certain cancers.

Effects on fertility and reproductive health.

Possible impact on sleep quality and brain function.

However, scientific consensus and regulatory bodies often highlight that the evidence linking EMFs to adverse health effects, especially at non-ionizing levels from everyday devices, remains inconclusive or lacks sufficient evidence to establish direct causal relationships.

Mitigation and Safety Measures:

Given the ongoing research and inconclusiveness, several precautionary measures and safety guidelines are recommended:

Minimize Exposure: Limiting exposure by keeping a distance from EMF sources, using hands-free devices for calls, and reducing screen time where feasible.

Follow Manufacturer Guidelines: Adhering to manufacturer recommendations for device usage and maintaining safe distances from high EMF sources.

Regulatory Standards: Governments and health organizations set safety standards and guidelines to limit exposure to EMFs, ensuring devices and technologies meet established safety thresholds.

Understanding EMFs involves acknowledging their presence in our environment while discerning the balance between potential risks and the benefits of modern technology. By staying informed, following safety guidelines, and supporting ongoing research, we can navigate the complex landscape of EMFs while making informed choices about our exposure and technology use.

CHAPTER 4: CHARGING UP: EXPLORING BATTERY TECHNOLOGY

INSIDE THE BATTERY: HOW IT STORES ENERGY

Batteries are the silent powerhouses that fuel our modern world, providing the energy necessary to power everything from smartphones to electric vehicles. Understanding how batteries store energy involves delving into the intricate processes occurring within these devices, revealing the fascinating science behind energy storage.

Composition and Structure:

At their core, batteries consist of one or more electrochemical cells, each containing three essential components:

Anode: The anode, typically made of graphite or lithium-based materials, serves as the electrode where the electrochemical reaction begins during charging or discharging.

Cathode: Complementing the anode, the cathode comprises materials such as lithium cobalt oxide or nickel manganese cobalt oxide. It acts as the electrode involved in the opposing reaction during charge and discharge cycles.

Electrolyte: The electrolyte, usually a liquid or gel substance containing lithium salts, facilitates the flow of ions between the anode and cathode while preventing direct contact between them.

Energy Storage Mechanism:

The process of storing energy within a battery occurs through electrochemical reactions between the anode and cathode. During charging, an external voltage applied to the battery forces lithium ions to move from the cathode to the anode through the electrolyte, where they're stored within the anode material.

This movement of ions causes a shift in the electrical potential of the battery, effectively storing electrical energy in the form of chemical potential energy within the anode material. Conversely, during discharge (when the battery powers a device), the stored ions flow back from the anode to the cathode through the electrolyte, producing an electric current that powers the connected device.

Ion Movement and Reaction:

The movement of ions within the battery involves a series of redox (reduction-oxidation) reactions. When the battery charges, lithium ions move from the cathode to the anode, where they are absorbed into the anode material. This absorption process involves the reduction of lithium ions into lithium atoms.

Upon discharge, as the battery powers a device, lithium ions move from the anode back to the cathode. During this process, the lithium atoms in the anode oxidize, releasing electrons that flow through the external circuit, generating electrical energy. Simultaneously, the lithium ions combine with electrons at the cathode, returning to their original state, ready for the next charge-discharge cycle.

Factors Influencing Battery Performance:

Several factors impact a battery's performance and overall efficiency:

Materials Used: The choice of materials for the anode, cathode, and electrolyte significantly influences a battery's capacity, voltage, and cycle life.

Charge Rate: Charging too quickly or at extreme temperatures can affect a battery's lifespan and safety.

Cycle Life: The number of charge-discharge cycles a battery can undergo before its capacity significantly diminishes.

Environmental Factors: Extreme temperatures, physical damage, and overcharging or deep discharging can degrade battery performance.

Understanding the science of energy storage within batteries illuminates the essential role they play in our daily lives. As research continues to innovate battery technologies, enhancing efficiency, capacity, and sustainability, these advancements pave the way for more powerful and environmentally friendly energy storage solutions that power the future of technology and transportation.

BATTERY LIFESPAN AND HEALTH IMPLICATIONS

Batteries are the lifeblood of our devices, powering everything from smartphones and laptops to electric vehicles. Understanding the factors that influence battery lifespan and the associated health implications is crucial for maximizing their longevity and maintaining optimal performance.

Factors Affecting Battery Lifespan:

Charge Cycles: A charge cycle refers to the process of charging a battery from 0% to 100%. Repeated charge-discharge cycles gradually degrade a battery's capacity. Lithium-ion batteries, common in many devices, have a limited number of charge cycles before their capacity diminishes significantly.

Temperature: Extreme temperatures, both hot and cold, can impact a battery's health. High temperatures accelerate chemical reactions within the battery, leading to quicker degradation. Similarly, very low temperatures can reduce a battery's efficiency temporarily.

Charge Levels: Keeping a battery at extreme charge levels (either fully charged or fully discharged) for extended periods can stress the battery and affect its long-term health. Avoiding prolonged storage at full charge or empty levels helps maintain battery health.

Charging Speed: Fast-charging technology, while convenient, can generate more heat within the battery, potentially impacting its longevity over time. Slower charging rates are generally considered less stressful for battery health.

Health Implications and Maintenance Tips:

Capacity Degradation: Over time, batteries lose their ability to hold a charge. This results in reduced runtime for devices and necessitates more frequent charging.

Increased Heat Generation: As batteries degrade, they tend to generate more heat during charging or usage, potentially affecting the device's performance and safety.

Reduced Overall Lifespan: Battery degradation eventually leads to a point where the battery's capacity becomes inadequate for practical use, requiring replacement or refurbishment.

Tips for Preserving Battery Health:

Avoid Extreme Temperatures: Keep devices within recommended temperature ranges to prevent accelerated battery degradation. Avoid leaving devices in direct sunlight or in overly cold environments for extended periods.

Moderate Charging Habits: Aim to keep batteries between 20% and 80% charge levels for optimal longevity. Avoid frequent full discharges or charges to 100% unless necessary.

Use Manufacturer-Recommended Chargers: Using official or compatible chargers recommended by the device manufacturer ensures proper voltage and current for safe and optimal charging.

Reduce Heat Exposure: Minimize factors that contribute to heat buildup in batteries, such as heavy usage during charging or using devices while they're charging.

Periodic Calibration: Some devices benefit from occasional full discharge and recharge cycles to recalibrate the battery gauge for accurate capacity readings.

Understanding the factors influencing battery lifespan and the associated health implications enables users to adopt practices that prolong battery life and optimize device performance. By following manufacturer guidelines, managing charging habits, and mitigating environmental stressors, individuals can maximize their battery's lifespan and maintain its health for sustained and efficient use.

SUSTAINABLE CHARGING SOLUTIONS

As society strives for greater sustainability and reduced environmental impact, the realm of charging solutions has seen significant advancements towards eco-friendly alternatives. Sustainable charging solutions encompass a range of technologies and practices aimed at minimizing energy consumption, utilizing renewable resources, and reducing carbon footprints in the process of powering our devices.

Renewable Energy-Powered Chargers:

Solar-Powered Chargers: These chargers harness solar energy through photovoltaic cells, converting sunlight into electrical power. Portable solar chargers provide a sustainable charging option, especially in outdoor settings or areas lacking traditional power sources.

Wind-Powered Chargers: Wind turbines generate electricity, which can be used to charge devices through wind-powered charging stations. These installations utilize wind energy to produce clean and renewable power for charging purposes.

Energy-Efficient Charging Practices:

Smart Charging Technology: Smart chargers incorporate technology that optimizes energy usage by adjusting charging rates based on device requirements. These chargers reduce energy wastage by delivering the precise amount of power needed for efficient charging.

Energy Management Systems: Implementing systems that monitor and manage power consumption, such as load balancing and demand-response strategies, ensures efficient use of electricity during charging processes.

Battery Innovations for Sustainability:

Solid-State Batteries: Research and development in solid-state battery technology aim to create batteries with higher energy densities, improved safety, and longer lifespans. These batteries have the potential to reduce reliance on traditional lithium-ion batteries and pave the way for more sustainable energy storage solutions.

Recyclable Battery Materials: Efforts to develop batteries using recyclable or sustainable materials reduce environmental impact. Designing batteries with easily recyclable components promotes circular economy principles, enabling the reuse of valuable materials.

Public Infrastructure and Initiatives:

Green Charging Stations: Governments and organizations worldwide are investing in green charging infrastructure. These stations often utilize renewable energy sources, providing clean and sustainable power for electric vehicles and devices.

Incentivizing Sustainable Charging: Policy measures, such as tax incentives or rebates for using renewable energy-powered chargers or energy-efficient devices, encourage individuals and businesses to adopt more sustainable charging practices.

Consumer Education and Behavioral Shifts:

Awareness and Education: Raising awareness about the environmental impact of traditional charging methods and promoting the benefits of sustainable alternatives encourage consumers to make greener choices.

Adopting Responsible Charging Habits: Encouraging users to adopt habits like unplugging chargers when not in use, using energy-efficient chargers, and avoiding overcharging contributes to reducing energy consumption and environmental impact.

The pursuit of sustainable charging solutions embodies a collective effort to minimize the carbon footprint associated with powering our devices. By embracing renewable energy sources, fostering innovation in battery technologies, and promoting energy-efficient practices, sustainable charging solutions play a pivotal role in advancing environmental stewardship while meeting the ever-growing demand for power in a greener and more sustainable manner.

CHAPTER 5: ELECTRIFYING EFFECTS: CHARGER IMPACT ON HUMAN PHYSIOLOGY

EFFECTS OF PROLONGED CHARGING DEVICE USAGE ON THE BODY

In today's digital age, the prolonged use of charging devices, such as smartphones, tablets, and laptops, has become a norm. While these devices offer immense convenience and connectivity, extended usage can potentially impact the body in various ways, affecting physical health and well-being.

1. Eye Strain and Visual Discomfort:

Prolonged screen time can lead to digital eye strain, also known as computer vision syndrome. Symptoms may include:

Eye discomfort

Dry or irritated eyes

Blurred vision

Headaches

Neck and shoulder pain due to poor posture

2. Disruption of Sleep Patterns:

Exposure to blue light emitted by screens, especially before bedtime, can disrupt the body's natural sleep-wake cycle. The suppression of melatonin, a hormone that regulates sleep, can lead to:

Difficulty falling asleep

Reduced quality of sleep

Disrupted circadian rhythm

3. Musculoskeletal Issues:

Poor posture while using charging devices for extended periods can contribute to musculoskeletal problems,

such as:

Neck strain (text neck)

Shoulder and back pain

Carpal tunnel syndrome or wrist discomfort due to repetitive movements

4. Mental and Emotional Impact:

Prolonged use of charging devices can also affect mental and emotional well-being:

Increased stress and anxiety, especially when exposed to negative content or excessive social media use

Reduced attention span and cognitive fatigue due to information overload

Impact on interpersonal relationships as excessive screen time may lead to reduced face-to-face interactions

Mitigating the Impact:

Take Regular Breaks: Follow the 20-20-20 rule—every 20 minutes, look at something 20 feet away for 20 seconds—to reduce eye strain.

Practice Good Posture: Maintain proper posture while using devices to alleviate strain on the neck, shoulders, and back.

Limit Screen Time: Set boundaries for screen usage, especially before bedtime, to improve sleep quality.

Use Blue Light Filters: Enable night mode or use blue light filters on devices to reduce exposure to blue light, particularly in the evenings.

Follow the 2-Hour Rule: Encourage breaks from screens, especially for children, by implementing a two-hour limit for continuous device usage.

Balancing the convenience of charging device usage with mindful practices is crucial to mitigate potential health impacts.

Implementing ergonomic habits, managing screen time, and prioritizing breaks contribute to maintaining physical health, mental well-being, and overall quality of life in this digitally-driven era.

NOT JUST VOLTAGE: EXPLORING PSYCHOLOGICAL EFFECTS

In our technologically immersed society, the psychological impact of charging devices extends beyond their functional utility. While these devices offer unparalleled connectivity and convenience, they also influence our psychological well-being in profound ways, shaping behaviors, emotions, and cognitive patterns.

1. Dependency and Addiction:

The allure of charging devices often leads to dependency and, in some cases, addiction. Constant notifications, social media interactions, and the urge to stay connected can foster a compulsive need to check devices frequently, leading to:

Increased anxiety when separated from devices

Difficulty in focusing on tasks without interruptions

The sensation of constantly needing to be 'plugged in' to the digital world

2. Social and Emotional Impact:

Charging devices profoundly affect our social and emotional spheres:

Social Comparison: Platforms like social media facilitate comparisons with others' lives, fostering feelings of inadequacy, envy, or fear of missing out (FOMO).

Impact on Relationships: Excessive device usage can impair real-world interactions, affecting the quality and depth of relationships with family and friends.

Emotional Well-being: Exposure to negative content or cyberbullying can impact mental health, leading to stress, depression, or feelings of isolation.

3. Cognitive Influence:

Charging devices have altered our cognitive processes:

Attention and Concentration: Constant notifications and the influx of information contribute to shortened attention spans, reduced concentration, and difficulty in sustaining focus.

Memory and Information Processing: The reliance on digital devices for information retrieval may diminish memory recall and affect critical thinking skills.

4. Sleep and Rest Disturbances:

Charging devices, particularly before bedtime, affect sleep patterns and overall rest:

Blue Light Impact: The blue light emitted by screens can disrupt the body's natural sleep cycle, delaying the onset of sleep and reducing the quality of rest.

Emotional Impact: Exposure to distressing or stimulating content before bed can evoke emotional responses that interfere with relaxation and sleep.

Mitigating Psychological Effects:

Digital Detoxes: Introduce periods of intentional disconnection from charging devices to restore mental clarity and reduce dependency.

Mindful Usage: Set boundaries and allocate specific times for device use, prioritizing real-world interactions and activities.

Limit Notifications: Disable non-essential notifications to reduce distractions and restore focus.

Establish Tech-Free Zones: Designate areas or times where charging devices are prohibited to promote face-to-face interactions and relaxation.

Understanding the multifaceted psychological impact of charging devices empowers individuals to adopt mindful practices, striking a balance between technological integration and mental well-being.

By cultivating a conscious relationship with these devices, individuals can harness their benefits while safeguarding against potential psychological repercussions.

POTENTIAL HEALTH RISKS ASSOCIATED WITH OVERCHARGING

Overcharging devices has become a common habit in our plugged-in society, where leaving devices connected to chargers for extended periods is a frequent occurrence. While modern technology incorporates safety features to prevent overcharging, prolonged charging beyond necessary levels may pose certain risks to both the device and the user's health.

1. Device Damage:

Battery Degradation: Overcharging can accelerate battery degradation. Continuous exposure to high voltage levels can cause stress on the battery, leading to reduced battery life and capacity over time.

Risk of Overheating: Prolonged charging generates excess heat within the device. Overheating not only damages the battery but can also impact other internal components, potentially leading to malfunctions or device failure.

2. Fire and Safety Hazards:

Increased Fire Risk: Overcharging can cause batteries to swell, leak, or, in extreme cases, catch fire or explode. Lithium-ion batteries, commonly used in devices, are sensitive to overcharging and can pose a fire hazard when damaged due to excessive voltage exposure.

3. Health Concerns:

Exposure to Harmful Chemicals: In rare instances of battery malfunctions due to overcharging, exposure to battery chemicals can occur. Contact with certain chemicals inside batteries can potentially cause skin irritation or burns.

Air Quality Concerns: If a device overheats or experiences a battery malfunction due to overcharging, it may release harmful chemicals or gases into the air, posing a risk to indoor air quality.

Mitigating Overcharging Risks:

Use Manufacturer-Approved Chargers: Ensure the use of chargers specifically designed for the device to prevent potential overcharging issues.

Unplug After Full Charge: Once devices reach a full charge, disconnect them from chargers to avoid continuous exposure to high voltage levels.

Avoid Overnight Charging: While many devices incorporate safety features, avoiding overnight charging reduces the duration of exposure to high voltage levels.

Monitor Battery Health: Utilize apps or device settings that display battery health to track the battery's condition and avoid unnecessary charging.

Replace Damaged Batteries: If a device's battery shows signs of damage or swelling, replace it promptly to prevent safety hazards.

Understanding the potential health and safety risks associated with overcharging devices underscores the importance of adopting responsible charging habits.

By adhering to recommended charging practices and being vigilant about battery health, individuals can minimize the risks of device damage, safety hazards, and potential health concerns stemming from overcharging.

CHAPTER 6: EMF EXPOSURE: UNDERSTANDING AND MANAGING RISKS

EXPLORING ELECTROMAGNETIC FIELDS (EMFS) AND HEALTH

Electromagnetic fields (EMFs) are ubiquitous in our modern world, generated by both natural sources and human-made technologies. EMFs encompass a spectrum of frequencies, and while they are an integral part of daily life, concerns persist about their potential impact on human health. Understanding EMFs and their association with health is essential for informed discourse on this complex subject.

Sources of Electromagnetic Fields:

Natural EMFs: Earth's magnetic field and cosmic rays from outer space generate natural EMFs that humans have been exposed to throughout evolution.

Man-Made EMFs: These include power lines, electrical wiring, household appliances, wireless devices (Wi-Fi, cell phones), and telecommunications infrastructure.

Types of EMFs:

Low-Frequency EMFs (ELF): Associated with power lines, electrical appliances, and transformers. ELF

EMFs have lower frequencies and are considered non-ionizing.

Radiofrequency EMFs (RF): Produced by wireless devices like cell phones, Wi-Fi routers, and microwave ovens. RF EMFs have higher frequencies and are also non-ionizing.

Health Considerations and Research:

The potential health effects of EMFs have been a subject of scientific inquiry and debate. Some studies suggest possible associations between EMF exposure and health concerns such as:

Cancer Risk: There have been investigations into a potential link between EMF exposure and certain types of cancers, especially childhood leukemia and brain tumors.

Electromagnetic Hypersensitivity (EHS): Some individuals report symptoms like headaches, fatigue, and sleep disturbances attributed to exposure to EMFs. However, scientific consensus has not established a causal relationship between EMFs and EHS.

Reproductive Health: Research has explored the impact of EMF exposure on reproductive health, including fertility and pregnancy outcomes. Findings have been inconclusive or conflicting.

Regulatory Guidelines and Safety Measures:

Safety Standards: Governments and international organizations set guidelines and safety limits for EMF exposure based on established research. These standards aim to protect the public from potential risks associated with EMFs.

Precautionary Measures: Some individuals choose to take precautionary steps such as minimizing exposure to EMFs, using devices at a distance, and employing shielding or protective measures.

The debate regarding the health effects of EMFs remains ongoing, with inconclusive or conflicting findings from scientific studies. While some research suggests potential associations with certain health concerns, regulatory standards aim to mitigate risks and ensure public safety.

More comprehensive and longitudinal studies are necessary to establish conclusive evidence about the relationship between EMFs and human health, allowing for informed decisions and policies regarding EMF exposure.

Measuring EMF Exposure

Measuring electromagnetic field (EMF) exposure is a crucial aspect of evaluating potential health risks associated with various sources of EMFs. Understanding how to assess and quantify EMF levels aids in determining exposure limits, ensuring compliance with safety guidelines, and addressing concerns related to human health. Here's an overview of the methods and considerations involved in measuring EMF exposure:

1. EMF Measurement Instruments:

Gaussmeters: These devices measure magnetic fields and are commonly used to assess low-frequency EMFs emitted by power lines, household appliances, and electrical equipment.

Electric Field Meters: Electric field meters gauge the strength of electric fields, especially in environments where electrical wiring or charged objects might emit such fields.

Radiofrequency Meters: Specifically designed for higher frequency EMFs like those emitted by cell phones, Wi-Fi routers, and other wireless devices, these meters quantify radiofrequency EMF exposure.

2. Measurement Units:

Magnetic Fields: Measured in units of tesla (T) or gauss (G), with typical exposure levels in milligauss (mg) for everyday environments.

Electric Fields: Units are volts per meter (V/m), measuring the electric field strength. For example, the human body is naturally exposed to electric fields from around 100 to 500 V/m.

Radiofrequency Fields: The unit of measurement is typically expressed in terms of power density (watts per square meter or W/m²) or specific absorption rate (SAR) for evaluating absorbed RF energy in the body.

3. Personal Exposure Assessments:

Wearable Monitors: Some devices are designed to be worn by individuals to track personal EMF exposure, providing real-time data on levels encountered throughout the day.

Dosimeters: These devices calculate cumulative exposure over time, providing a comprehensive assessment of EMF exposure within a specific period.

4. Environmental Surveys and Site Assessments:

Area Monitoring: Conducting measurements across different locations to identify areas with elevated EMF levels or hotspots.

Occupational Exposure Assessments: Evaluating EMF levels in work environments, especially for occupations involving exposure to higher EMF sources like power plants or telecommunication facilities.

Safety Considerations and Guidelines:

Regulatory Standards: Governments and health organizations establish safety limits and guidelines for EMF exposure based on scientific research. These standards aim to protect the public from potential health risks associated with EMFs.

Precautionary Measures: Despite the absence of conclusive evidence linking EMFs to adverse health effects, some individuals choose to minimize exposure by practicing prudent habits, such as maintaining distance from EMF sources or limiting screen time.

Measuring EMF exposure involves utilizing specialized instruments and techniques to assess the intensity of electromagnetic fields in various environments.

While regulatory guidelines exist to ensure safety, ongoing research continues to refine our understanding of EMFs and their potential impact on human health, enabling informed decisions and policies regarding EMF exposure.

MITIGATING EMF EXPOSURE RISKS

As technology continues to permeate every aspect of our lives, concerns about electromagnetic field (EMF) exposure have gained attention due to their potential health implications. While conclusive evidence on EMF-related health risks remains inconclusive, adopting prudent practices to minimize exposure is a proactive approach toward safer technology use. Here are strategies to mitigate EMF exposure risks:

1. Maintain Distance from EMF Sources:

Keep Devices at a Distance: Maintain a reasonable distance between the body and devices emitting EMFs, such as cell phones, laptops, and routers, especially during prolonged usage.

Reduce Use of Wireless Devices: Minimize direct contact by using speakerphone or wired headsets while making calls or texting instead of holding devices close to the body.

2. Use EMF-Shielding Products:

EMF-Protective Cases or Shields: Consider using protective cases or shields specifically designed to reduce EMF exposure from devices.

EMF-Blocking Materials: Certain fabrics and materials claim to block or reduce EMF radiation, providing shielding when placed between the body and devices.

3. Limit Screen Time and Wireless Connections:

Implement Screen Time Boundaries: Reduce overall screen time, especially for children, and encourage breaks from devices to minimize continuous EMF exposure.

Use Wired Connections: Opt for wired connections (Ethernet cables) rather than wireless connections (Wi-Fi) when feasible to reduce exposure to radiofrequency EMFs.

4. Optimize Device Usage Habits:

Disable Non-Essential Wireless Functions: Turn off Wi-Fi, Bluetooth, and cellular data when not in use to reduce unnecessary EMF emissions from devices.

Avoid Sleeping with Devices: Refrain from keeping charging devices close to the body, especially during sleep, to minimize prolonged EMF exposure.

5. Create Low-EMF Environments:

Design EMF-Safe Spaces: Organize living and work environments by arranging furniture and devices in a way that reduces close contact and exposure to EMFs.

Reduce EMF Sources: Limit the number of electronic devices in close proximity and consider relocating sources like routers away from frequently occupied areas.

6. Educate and Stay Informed:

Stay Updated with Research: Keep abreast of scientific studies and regulatory guidelines on EMF exposure to make informed decisions about technology usage.

Raise Awareness: Educate yourself and others about potential EMF exposure risks and strategies to minimize them without causing undue alarm.

7. Seek Professional Assessments:

EMF Assessments: Consider professional assessments of EMF levels in your home or workspace to identify potential high-exposure areas and implement appropriate mitigation measures.

While the scientific community continues to study EMF exposure and its potential health effects, adopting practical and precautionary measures to reduce exposure can contribute to a safer technology environment. Striking a balance between utilizing technology and minimizing EMF exposure risks is essential for informed and responsible technology usage in today's connected world.

CHAPTER 7: THE CHARGING RITUAL: HEALTHY CHARGING HABITS

ESTABLISHING HEALTHY CHARGING PRACTICES

In our digitally driven world, where smartphones, tablets, laptops, and various gadgets have become indispensable, adopting healthy charging practices is crucial for maintaining device performance and ensuring personal safety. Balancing convenience with responsible charging habits can prolong battery life, mitigate potential risks, and optimize overall device usage. Here are key strategies to establish healthy charging practices:

1. Use Manufacturer-Approved Chargers:

Genuine Chargers: Utilize chargers provided by the device manufacturer or certified third-party chargers to ensure compatibility and safe charging.

2. Avoid Overcharging:

Unplug After Full Charge: Disconnect devices from chargers once they reach a full charge to prevent overcharging, which can stress the battery and reduce its lifespan.

3. Monitor Charging Duration:

Time Charging Cycles: Aim for shorter charging durations by plugging in devices when necessary and unplugging them promptly upon reaching sufficient charge levels.

4. Mindful Charging Environments:

Avoid Extreme Temperatures: Charging devices in excessively hot or cold environments can impact battery health. Opt for moderate temperature settings for optimal charging conditions.

5. Optimize Charging Frequency:

Partial Charging vs. Full Discharge: Lithium-ion batteries, common in many devices, benefit from frequent partial charges instead of complete discharge cycles, which can strain the battery.

6. Prevent Physical Damage:

Protect Charging Cables: Avoid bending or twisting charging cables excessively and handle them gently to prevent damage, ensuring safe and consistent charging.

7. Implement Charging Time Restrictions:

Avoid Overnight Charging: While many devices incorporate safety features, charging devices overnight exposes batteries to unnecessary stress. Charge devices during waking hours to monitor charging progress.

8. Consider Battery Health Indicators:

Utilize Device Settings: Some devices offer battery health indicators or optimization settings. Monitor battery health and use these features to maintain optimal charging levels.

9. Invest in Smart Charging Accessories:

Smart Power Strips: Use power strips equipped with timers or surge protection features to control charging times and safeguard devices against power surges.

10. Educate and Promote Responsible Charging:

Share Guidelines: Educate family members, especially children and teens, about responsible charging practices to instill good habits and prolong device lifespan.

By integrating these healthy charging practices into your routine, you can ensure the longevity of your devices, optimize battery health, and reduce the risk of potential hazards associated with improper charging habits. Balancing convenience with mindful charging habits fosters a safer and more sustainable approach to utilizing technology in our daily lives.

BEST PRACTICES FOR SAFE AND EFFICIENT CHARGING

Charging electronic devices efficiently and safely is essential for maintaining device health, maximizing battery lifespan, and ensuring personal safety. Implementing best practices not only optimizes charging but also minimizes risks associated with overcharging, overheating, and potential hazards. Here are key strategies for safe and efficient charging:

1. Use Genuine Chargers and Cables:

Manufacturer-Approved Accessories: Utilize original chargers and cables provided by the device manufacturer or certified third-party accessories to ensure compatibility and safe charging.

2. Check Charging Equipment:

Inspect Regularly: Periodically examine chargers, cables, and power outlets for signs of wear, fraying, or damage. Replace damaged equipment promptly to avoid safety hazards.

3. Charge in Moderate Temperatures:

Avoid Extreme Conditions: Charge devices in environments with moderate temperatures. Extremes in temperature, both hot and cold, can affect battery health and charging efficiency.

4. Unplug After Full Charge:

Prevent Overcharging: Disconnect devices from chargers once they reach full charge to prevent overcharging, which can stress the battery and diminish its lifespan.

5. Practice Partial Charging:

Avoid Complete Discharge: Frequent partial charging is preferable to full discharge cycles for lithium-ion batteries. Avoid letting batteries drain completely before recharging.

6. Avoid Charging on Soft Surfaces:

Use Stable Surfaces: Charge devices on stable and flat surfaces to allow for proper ventilation and prevent overheating, minimizing potential fire hazards.

7. Mindful Charging Times:

Charge During Wakeful Hours: Refrain from overnight charging whenever possible. Charging during waking hours allows monitoring and prevents extended exposure to fully charged states.

8. Enable Battery Health Features:

Utilize Device Settings: Some devices offer battery optimization features or health indicators. Utilize these settings to maintain battery health and prolong lifespan.

9. Limit Fast Charging Practices:

Use Moderately: Fast-charging technology can generate more heat and stress the battery. Limit fast-charging practices to when necessary to preserve battery health.

10. Educate and Promote Safe Charging:

Share Knowledge: Educate family members, especially children and elderly individuals, about safe charging practices to prevent accidents and ensure responsible usage.

By incorporating these best practices into your routine, you can optimize the efficiency of charging electronic devices while safeguarding against potential hazards and maximizing the lifespan of batteries. Responsible charging habits contribute to a safer and more sustainable approach to utilizing technology in our daily lives.

IMPORTANCE OF PROPER CHARGING ETIQUETTE

In today's technology-centric world, where electronic devices are an integral part of our daily lives, understanding and practicing proper charging etiquette is paramount. Establishing respectful and responsible charging habits not only ensures the safety and longevity of devices but also contributes to energy efficiency and promotes a mindful approach to technology usage. Here's why proper charging etiquette is crucial:

1. Device Safety and Longevity:

Preventing Hazards: Proper charging practices minimize the risk of potential hazards such as overheating, electrical fires, and damage to devices caused by faulty chargers or cables.

Extending Battery Life: Adhering to optimal charging methods, such as avoiding overcharging and extreme temperatures, preserves battery health and extends the lifespan of electronic devices.

2. Energy Conservation and Efficiency:

Reducing Energy Waste: Unplugging devices after reaching a full charge prevents unnecessary energy consumption, contributing to energy conservation and reducing utility costs.

Minimizing Environmental Impact: Responsible charging habits translate to reduced energy usage, aligning with sustainable practices and contributing to a smaller environmental footprint.

3. Safety and Fire Prevention:

Preventing Fire Hazards: Charging devices on stable surfaces and avoiding charging on flammable materials helps prevent overheating and potential fire hazards, ensuring personal and property safety.

4. Cultivating Responsible Technology Use:

Educating and Raising Awareness: Emphasizing proper charging etiquette educates individuals, especially children and teens, about responsible technology usage and safety measures.

Promoting Consideration: Encouraging mindful charging habits fosters consideration for shared charging spaces, allowing fair access to charging outlets for all individuals.

5. Maximizing Public Charging Spaces:

Ensuring Accessibility: Adhering to proper charging etiquette in public spaces ensures that charging outlets remain available to all users, preventing unnecessary wait times or inconvenience.

6. Cultural and Social Norms:

Establishing Norms: Integrating proper charging practices into societal norms fosters a culture of consideration, responsibility, and respect for shared resources.

Proper charging etiquette goes beyond mere technical guidelines; it encompasses a conscientious approach to utilizing technology while prioritizing safety, energy efficiency, and responsible device usage. By adopting and promoting these practices, individuals contribute to a safer, more sustainable, and considerate technological landscape, ensuring the well-being of devices, users, and the environment alike.

CHAPTER 8: INNOVATIONS IN CHARGER TECHNOLOGY

CUTTING-EDGE CHARGING SOLUTIONS AND FUTURE TRENDS

The world of charging solutions is continuously evolving, driven by innovation, sustainability, and the quest for enhanced efficiency. As technology advances, new methodologies, and breakthroughs in charging solutions are transforming how we power our devices. Here's an exploration of cutting-edge charging solutions and future trends shaping the landscape:

1. Wireless Charging Advancements:

Extended Range Wireless Charging: Innovations in wireless charging technology are extending the range and efficiency of wireless power transfer, allowing devices to charge even at a distance from charging pads or stations.

Fast Wireless Charging: Ongoing research aims to improve the speed of wireless charging, delivering rapid and efficient power transfer without the need for physical connections.

2. Rapid Advancements in Battery Technology:

Solid-State Batteries: The development of solid-state batteries promises higher energy density, improved safety, and faster charging capabilities compared to traditional lithium-ion batteries.

Lithium-Sulfur Batteries: Exploration of lithium-sulfur batteries presents potential breakthroughs in higher energy densities, lower costs, and reduced environmental impact compared to existing battery technologies.

3. Energy Harvesting and Sustainable Solutions:

Solar-Powered Chargers: Advancements in solar charging technology continue to make solar-powered chargers more efficient and practical for powering devices, especially in remote or outdoor settings.

Kinetic Energy Harvesting: Devices capable of harvesting kinetic energy from motion or movement offer alternative ways to power smaller gadgets and wearables, reducing dependency on traditional charging methods.

4. Fast-Charging Innovations:

Ultra-Fast Charging: Research into ultra-fast charging solutions aims to reduce charging times significantly, enabling devices to reach full charge within minutes instead of hours.

Graphene-Based Charging: Graphene-based supercapacitors show potential for faster charging rates, increased energy density, and enhanced durability compared to conventional batteries.

5. Eco-Friendly Charging Infrastructure:

Green Charging Stations: Integration of renewable energy sources, such as solar or wind power, into public charging infrastructure promotes sustainable and eco-friendly charging solutions for electric vehicles and devices.

6. Integration of Smart and Adaptive Charging:

AI-Powered Charging Systems: Implementation of artificial intelligence (AI) in charging systems enables adaptive and optimized charging patterns based on usage habits, battery health, and energy availability.

Smart Grid Integration: Integration of charging systems with smart grids facilitates efficient energy distribution and charging optimization, enhancing overall energy management.

7. Bidirectional Charging and Energy Sharing:

V2G Technology: Vehicle-to-Grid (V2G) technology allows electric vehicles to not only charge from the grid but also feed stored energy back into the grid, contributing to grid stability and energy sharing.

Cutting-edge charging solutions and emerging trends signify a future where charging becomes faster, more efficient, and increasingly sustainable. These advancements hold the promise of revolutionizing how we power our devices, shaping a more connected, eco-friendly, and efficient technological landscape.

As research and innovation continue to propel the field forward, the evolution of charging solutions will undoubtedly play a pivotal role in shaping our technological future.

WIRELESS CHARGING: PROS, CONS, AND HEALTH CONSIDERATIONS

Wireless charging technology has revolutionized how we power our devices, offering convenience and eliminating the need for tangled cables. However, like any technology, it comes with its advantages, drawbacks, and health considerations. Here's an exploration of the pros, cons, and health aspects associated with wireless charging:

Pros of Wireless Charging:

Convenience and Ease of Use: Simply placing a device on a charging pad or stand eliminates the hassle of plugging and unplugging cables, providing a seamless and effortless charging experience.

Reduced Wear and Tear: Frequent plugging and unplugging of charging cables can cause wear and tear on ports and cables. Wireless charging minimizes this issue, potentially prolonging the lifespan of devices.

Versatility and Compatibility: Wireless charging is becoming increasingly compatible with various devices, from smartphones and tablets to wearables and even some laptops, offering versatility in charging options.

Aesthetic Appeal: Wireless charging pads or stands can contribute to a clutter-free and visually appealing charging setup without the presence of numerous cables.

Cons of Wireless Charging:

Slower Charging Speeds: In comparison to wired charging, wireless charging tends to be slower, especially when using standard charging pads, which may prolong the time needed to reach a full charge.

Heat Generation: Wireless charging can generate more heat compared to wired charging. This excess heat may affect battery lifespan and device performance over time.

Limited Mobility While Charging: Devices must remain in close proximity to the charging pad, limiting mobility during charging. Picking up or using the device while charging is less convenient than with a plugged-in cable.

Efficiency Losses: Energy transfer in wireless charging can experience efficiency losses, leading to wasted energy, albeit minimal, during the charging process.

Health Considerations:

Electromagnetic Exposure: Wireless charging emits electromagnetic fields (EMFs) during operation. While most research indicates that typical exposure levels are safe, some individuals may prefer to minimize prolonged exposure to EMFs as a precaution.

Heat Emission: Excessive heat generated during wireless charging may potentially affect battery health and, in rare cases, could cause discomfort if devices become excessively hot.

Wireless charging offers undeniable convenience and aesthetics, making it a popular choice for many users. However, slower charging speeds, potential efficiency losses, and concerns about heat generation and electromagnetic exposure are important factors to consider. Users should weigh the convenience against the potential drawbacks and health considerations to determine whether wireless charging is the right choice for their needs and preferences.

As technology continues to evolve, advancements in wireless charging may address some of these drawbacks, making it an even more viable and efficient charging option.

ECO-FRIENDLY CHARGING INNOVATIONS

In an era increasingly focused on sustainability, the evolution of charging technologies has witnessed a surge in eco-friendly innovations aimed at reducing environmental impact and promoting energy efficiency. These advancements are revolutionizing the way we power our devices, vehicles, and homes. Here's an exploration of some pioneering eco-friendly charging innovations:

1. Solar-Powered Charging Solutions:

Solar Panels for Devices: Integration of solar panels into charging devices allows users to harness renewable solar energy to power smartphones, tablets, and other gadgets, especially in outdoor settings.

Solar Chargers for Electric Vehicles: Advancements in solar-powered car charging stations enable electric vehicles (EVs) to harness clean energy, reducing reliance on grid electricity.

2. Sustainable Materials in Charging Equipment:

Biodegradable Charging Accessories: The use of biodegradable or recyclable materials in manufacturing charging cables, adapters, and charging stations reduces environmental impact.

3. Energy Harvesting Technologies:

Kinetic Energy Harvesting: Devices that capture and convert kinetic energy from movement or motion into electrical power offer an innovative way to charge wearables and small gadgets.

Thermoelectric Generators: Utilizing temperature differences to generate electricity, thermoelectric generators can potentially power small devices and sensors in eco-friendly ways.

4. Green Charging Infrastructure:

Renewable-Powered Charging Stations: Integrating renewable energy sources like solar or wind power into public charging infrastructure promotes sustainable charging solutions for electric vehicles.

Smart Grid Integration: Connecting charging systems to smart grids allows for optimized energy distribution, peak-time charging, and utilization of clean energy sources.

5. Eco-Friendly Battery Technologies:

Recyclable Batteries: Developing batteries with materials that are easier to recycle or repurpose reduces waste and supports circular economy principles.

Low-Impact Battery Chemistries: Exploring battery technologies with reduced environmental impact, such as lithium-iron-phosphate batteries, aims to minimize resource depletion and ecological footprint.

6. Energy-Efficient Charging Algorithms:

AI-Powered Charging Optimization: Implementing artificial intelligence (AI) in charging systems enables intelligent algorithms to optimize charging patterns based on energy availability and demand.

7. Bidirectional Charging and Grid Integration:

Vehicle-to-Grid (V2G) Technology: EVs equipped with V2G capabilities can not only charge from the grid but also supply stored energy back to the grid, contributing to grid stability and energy balance.

Eco-friendly charging innovations are propelling a transition towards sustainable power solutions, offering a promising pathway to reduce reliance on non-renewable energy sources and minimize environmental impact. As these technologies continue to evolve and integrate into our daily lives, they play a pivotal role in shaping a more sustainable future by fostering energy efficiency, reducing carbon footprints, and promoting responsible energy consumption.

CHAPTER 9: CHARGER SAFETY AND REGULATIONS

ENSURING CHARGER SAFETY STANDARDS

Chargers play a pivotal role in powering our electronic devices, but their safety and adherence to standards are crucial to prevent potential hazards and ensure user safety. Here's an overview of the importance of charger safety standards and measures to ensure their compliance:

Why Charger Safety Standards Matter:

Preventing Electrical Hazards: Adherence to safety standards prevents electrical hazards like short circuits, overcharging, overheating, and electrical fires that can result from faulty chargers.

Device Protection: Safe chargers help protect devices from damage caused by irregular voltage, excessive current, or inadequate insulation, preserving the lifespan and functionality of gadgets.

User Safety: Ensuring safety standards reduces the risk of electrical shocks, burns, or injuries to users that may occur due to substandard or counterfeit chargers.

Key Measures to Ensure Charger Safety Standards:

Certification and Compliance:

CE, UL, FCC Certification: Look for chargers with certifications such as CE (Conformité Européenne), UL (Underwriters Laboratories), or FCC (Federal Communications Commission), indicating compliance with safety standards.

Genuine Accessories:

Manufacturer-Supplied Chargers: Use original chargers supplied by device manufacturers or reputable third-party chargers designed specifically for the device model to ensure compatibility and safety.

Visual Inspection:

Check for Physical Damage: Inspect chargers and cables regularly for signs of wear, fraying, or exposed wires. Damaged chargers should be replaced immediately to avoid safety risks.

Purchase from Reputable Sources:

Avoid Counterfeit Chargers: Purchase chargers from trusted retailers or authorized distributors to reduce the risk of buying counterfeit or substandard products that may not meet safety standards.

Proper Usage Practices:

Avoid Overloading Outlets: Refrain from connecting multiple devices to a single outlet or using low-quality extension cords to prevent overheating and potential fire hazards.

Follow Manufacturer Recommendations:

Adhere to Manufacturer Guidelines: Follow device-specific charging instructions and recommended charger ratings to ensure safe and optimal charging.

Public Awareness and Education:

Educate Users: Raise awareness among consumers about the importance of using safe chargers and recognizing potential risks associated with substandard charging accessories.

Adherence to charger safety standards is paramount to safeguarding devices, users, and properties from potential electrical hazards. Utilizing certified and genuine chargers, conducting regular inspections, and fostering awareness among users about safe charging practices are instrumental in ensuring compliance with safety standards. By prioritizing safety in the selection and usage of chargers, individuals can mitigate risks and maintain a secure charging environment for their electronic devices.

GLOBAL REGULATIONS AND COMPLIANCE

In today's interconnected world, global regulations and compliance standards play a pivotal role in ensuring product safety, quality, and uniformity across international markets. These regulations are essential for protecting consumers, preserving environmental sustainability, and fostering fair trade practices. Here's an overview of the significance and impact of global regulations and compliance:

Importance of Global Regulations:

Consumer Protection: Regulations set minimum safety and quality standards for products, safeguarding consumers from potential hazards, substandard goods, and misleading claims.

Environmental Conservation: Compliance with environmental regulations reduces the ecological impact of products, ensuring responsible sourcing, manufacturing, and disposal practices.

Fair Trade Practices: Regulations promote fair competition, preventing monopolies, price fixing, and unfair market practices, fostering a level playing field for businesses.

Key Aspects of Global Regulations and Compliance:

Standardization Bodies:

ISO (International Organization for Standardization): ISO develops and publishes international standards that ensure product quality, safety, and efficiency across industries.

IEC (International Electrotechnical Commission): IEC sets standards for electrical and electronic technologies, including safety requirements for electronic devices and chargers.

Product Certification and Compliance Marks:

CE Marking (Conformité Européenne): The CE mark indicates compliance with European Union (EU) health, safety, and environmental protection standards for products sold within the EU.

FCC (Federal Communications Commission): In the United States, the FCC certification ensures electromagnetic compatibility and compliance with radio frequency regulations.

Industry-Specific Regulations:

Charger Safety Standards: Regulations govern charger safety, efficiency, and electromagnetic compatibility, ensuring compliance with safety measures and performance criteria.

Trade Agreements and Regional Regulations:

Trade Blocks: Regional trade agreements, such as the European Union's directives or North American Free Trade Agreement (NAFTA), establish common regulations and standards within specific economic zones.

Challenges and Considerations:

Divergent Standards: Varied regulatory requirements across regions or countries can pose challenges for manufacturers aiming to comply with multiple standards simultaneously.

Rapid Technological Advancements: Regulating emerging technologies like wireless charging, AI, and IoT devices requires adaptable frameworks to keep pace with innovation.

Enforcement and Compliance Monitoring: Ensuring consistent adherence to regulations globally necessitates robust monitoring mechanisms and cooperation between regulatory authorities.

Global regulations and compliance frameworks are instrumental in maintaining product safety, quality, and environmental sustainability on a worldwide scale. Harmonizing standards, enhancing collaboration between regulatory bodies, and adapting to technological advancements remain crucial for fostering a secure, fair, and standardized global marketplace. Compliance with these regulations not only ensures consumer safety but also facilitates international trade while fostering innovation and sustainable development.

CONSUMER RIGHTS AND CHARGER SAFETY

In the realm of technological advancements, consumer rights play a vital role in ensuring the safety, quality, and reliability of products, particularly concerning charger safety. Empowering consumers with rights and information is essential for safeguarding their interests and promoting accountability among manufacturers and sellers. Here's an exploration of consumer rights concerning charger safety:

1. Right to Safety and Quality:

Consumers have the fundamental right to expect products, including chargers, to be safe for use and compliant with established safety standards to prevent hazards or risks.

2. Right to Information and Transparency:

Consumers are entitled to clear and accurate information about charger specifications, safety features, certifications, and compliance with relevant safety standards.

3. Right to Redress and Compensation:

In case of defective or unsafe chargers causing harm or damage, consumers have the right to seek compensation, refunds, repairs, or replacements as per consumer protection laws.

4. Right to Fair Practices and Accountability:

Consumers have the right to fair trade practices and expect manufacturers and sellers to adhere to safety standards, ensuring accountability for product safety and quality.

Key Aspects of Charger Safety in Relation to Consumer Rights:

Certification and Compliance:

Consumers should look for charger certifications (e.g., CE, UL, FCC) indicating compliance with safety standards, ensuring product safety and reliability.

Transparency in Product Information:

Manufacturers should provide comprehensive information on charger specifications, including input/output ratings, compatibility, and safety features, aiding informed consumer decisions.

Recall and Safety Alerts:

Consumers have the right to be informed about charger recalls or safety alerts issued by manufacturers or regulatory authorities to address potential safety concerns promptly.

Accessibility to Redress Mechanisms:

Access to complaint resolution systems, customer support, and avenues for seeking redress in case of safety issues with chargers is essential to uphold consumer rights.

Consumer Education and Awareness:

Empowering consumers with knowledge about charger safety, compliance standards, and red flags for unsafe chargers is crucial to enable informed purchasing decisions.

Consumer rights regarding charger safety encompass a broad spectrum of protections, including the right to safety, information, redress, and fair practices. Upholding these rights requires collaboration between regulatory bodies, manufacturers, sellers, and informed consumer participation. Ensuring charger safety aligns with consumer rights, promoting accountability and transparency in the marketplace, ultimately safeguarding consumers from potential hazards and ensuring their well-being.

CHAPTER 10: MINDFUL TECH USE: BALANCING SCREEN TIME AND HEALTH

UNDERSTANDING SCREEN TIME AND ITS IMPACT

In the digital age, screen time, referring to the duration spent using digital devices such as smartphones, computers, tablets, and TVs, has become an integral part of daily life. While technology offers numerous benefits, excessive screen time can impact various aspects of health and well-being. Here's an exploration of screen time and its effects:

1. Impact on Physical Health:

Sedentary Behavior: Excessive screen time often leads to a sedentary lifestyle, contributing to a lack of physical activity and increased risk of obesity and related health issues.

Eye Strain and Discomfort: Prolonged exposure to screens may cause eye strain, dry eyes, headaches, and discomfort, known as computer vision syndrome.

Sleep Disturbances: Excessive screen time, especially before bedtime, can disrupt sleep patterns due to the blue light emitted by screens, affecting the quality and duration of sleep.

2. Effects on Mental and Emotional Well-being:

Impact on Mental Health: Excessive screen time, particularly on social media platforms, may contribute to stress, anxiety, depression, and reduced self-esteem, influenced by comparison and cyberbullying.

Social Interactions: Excessive reliance on digital communication can lead to reduced face-to-face interactions, potentially affecting social skills and relationships.

Addictive Behaviors: Excessive use of screens, particularly in gaming or social media, may lead to addictive behaviors and dependency, impacting mental health and productivity.

3. Cognitive Impacts:

Attention and Cognitive Function: Excessive screen time, especially in children, may affect attention span, cognitive development, and the ability to focus on tasks.

Educational Impact: While technology aids learning, excessive screen time without moderation or guidance can impede learning and academic performance.

Strategies for Managing Screen Time:

Set Screen Time Limits: Establish designated periods for screen use, incorporating breaks to reduce prolonged exposure.

Create Tech-Free Zones: Designate areas like bedrooms or dining areas as tech-free zones to promote family interaction and quality time.

Encourage Physical Activity: Balance screen time with outdoor activities, exercise, hobbies, and other non-screen-related pursuits.

Implement Screen Time Guidelines: For children, follow age-appropriate screen time guidelines recommended by pediatric associations.

Practice Digital Detox: Periodically disconnect from screens to recharge mentally and emotionally, promoting mindfulness and reducing dependency.

Understanding the impact of screen time on various aspects of health and well-being is essential for individuals and families.

Balancing the benefits of technology with moderation and healthy screen time habits is key to promoting a balanced lifestyle and mitigating potential adverse effects on physical, mental, and emotional health. Striking a healthy balance in screen time usage contributes to overall well-being and a more fulfilling life.

STRATEGIES FOR BALANCING TECH USE AND WELLNESS

In today's digitally driven world, striking a healthy balance between technology usage and overall well-being is essential for maintaining a harmonious lifestyle. Here are effective strategies to foster a balanced approach to tech use and prioritize wellness:

1. Set Boundaries and Establish Tech-Free Times:

Designate Screen-Free Hours: Create specific time slots, such as during meals or before bedtime, dedicated to disconnecting from devices to promote family interaction and better sleep quality.

2. Practice Mindful Technology Use:

Mindful Screen Engagement: Be intentional about technology use, focusing on productive tasks or activities rather than mindless scrolling or constant notifications.

3. Prioritize Real-Life Connections:

Face-to-Face Interactions: Nurture in-person relationships by scheduling regular meetups, outings, or gatherings with friends and family to maintain meaningful connections.

4. Implement Digital Detox Periods:

Scheduled Breaks: Plan regular breaks from technology, whether it's a day or a weekend, to detoxify from screens and engage in offline activities like hobbies, reading, or outdoor pursuits.

5. Utilize Tech for Wellness:

Wellness Apps and Tools: Explore apps focusing on mindfulness, meditation, fitness, or mental health to leverage technology for enhancing well-being rather than solely for entertainment.

6. Create Tech-Free Zones or Activities:

Designated Spaces: Establish areas in your home or specific activities (e.g., yoga, meditation) where technology is not allowed, fostering an environment conducive to relaxation and focus.

7. Set Screen Time Limits:

Use Parental Controls: For children, implement parental controls or screen time management features to regulate and monitor their technology usage.

8. Engage in Physical Activity:

Balance with Exercise: Dedicate time to physical activities, workouts, or outdoor exercises to counterbalance sedentary screen time and promote physical wellness.

9. Foster Mental Well-being:

Limit Exposure to Negative Content: Be mindful of the content consumed online and consider limiting exposure to negative or stressful information to protect mental health.

10. Lead by Example:

Model Healthy Tech Habits: Demonstrate balanced technology use to children or family members by following similar guidelines and being mindful of your own screen time.

11. Seek Support and Connection:

Community Engagement: Engage in communities or groups with similar interests offline to foster connections and reduce dependency on technology for social interaction.

Striking a balance between technology use and wellness involves conscious effort, setting boundaries, and embracing a mindful approach to screen time. By incorporating these strategies into daily routines, individuals can cultivate a healthier relationship with technology, promote overall wellness, and enjoy a more fulfilling and balanced lifestyle. Regularly reassessing and adjusting these strategies can help maintain a harmonious balance between tech use and personal well-being.

ENCOURAGING MINDFUL TECHNOLOGY HABITS

In a digitally immersive world, fostering mindful technology habits is essential for cultivating a healthier relationship with digital devices. Practicing mindfulness in technology use involves being intentional, aware, and purposeful in our interactions with screens and digital platforms. Here are strategies to encourage mindful technology habits:

1. Set Intentions and Goals:

Define Purposeful Use: Determine clear objectives for using technology, whether it's for work, learning, communication, or leisure, and align screen time with these intentions.

2. Create Awareness and Conscious Engagement:

Practice Self-Awareness: Regularly check in with yourself about how you're using technology, noticing habits, emotions, and reactions related to screen time.

Mindful Check-ins: Take brief pauses during technology use to assess your focus, posture, and mental state, ensuring a mindful and present experience.

3. Implement Tech-Free Rituals:

Morning and Evening Rituals: Start or end the day without immediate screen exposure by incorporating tech-free activities like meditation, journaling, or reading.

4. Establish Boundaries and Limits:

Set Time Limits: Allocate specific durations for screen time and establish boundaries to avoid excessive or aimless browsing, especially during leisure hours.

5. Practice Mindful Consumption:

Curate Content Mindfully: Consume content intentionally by selecting valuable, informative, or inspiring material, minimizing exposure to content that provokes stress or negativity.

6. Embrace Digital Detox Periods:

Scheduled Breaks: Plan periodic breaks or tech-free days to disconnect from screens entirely, allowing mental rejuvenation and engagement in offline activities.

7. Engage in One Task at a Time:

Focus on Single Tasks: Avoid multitasking on multiple screens or devices, focusing on one task at a time to enhance concentration and productivity.

8. Prioritize Human Connections:

Quality Interactions: Prioritize face-to-face conversations and real-life interactions over virtual communication, fostering deeper and more meaningful connections.

9. Practice Gratitude and Mindfulness:

Gratitude Practice: Cultivate a sense of gratitude for the opportunities and benefits technology provides while being mindful of its limitations and potential pitfalls.

10. Reflect and Adjust Habits:

Regular Reflection: Periodically reflect on your technology habits, assessing their impact on mental health, productivity, and overall well-being. Adjust habits accordingly.

Encouraging mindful technology habits involves consciously engaging with digital devices while prioritizing awareness, intentionality, and balance. By adopting these strategies, individuals can foster a healthier relationship with technology, promoting mental clarity, emotional well-being, and a more fulfilling and mindful approach to life in the digital age. Cultivating mindful technology habits not only enhances productivity and focus but also supports a more conscious and balanced lifestyle.

CHAPTER 11: THE FUTURE OF CHARGERS AND WELLNESS

EMERGING TRENDS IN CHARGER TECHNOLOGY

Charger technology continues to evolve rapidly, driven by innovation, efficiency, and the demand for faster, safer, and more versatile charging solutions. Emerging trends in charger technology are revolutionizing how we power our devices, paving the way for more advanced and convenient charging experiences. Here's an exploration of some cutting-edge trends:

1. Wireless Charging Advancements:

Extended Range Charging: Ongoing research focuses on enhancing the distance and efficiency of wireless power transfer, enabling charging over longer distances without physical contact.

Fast Wireless Charging: Advancements aim to boost the speed of wireless charging, reducing charging times significantly to provide rapid power transfer without compromising efficiency.

2. GaN (Gallium Nitride) Chargers:

Efficiency and Compact Design: GaN chargers, known for their higher efficiency and smaller footprint compared to traditional silicon-based chargers, are gaining popularity for faster and more compact charging solutions.

3. USB-C Power Delivery (PD):

Universal Compatibility and Fast Charging: USB-C PD technology offers universal compatibility across devices and provides fast-charging capabilities, supporting higher power outputs for various gadgets.

4. Bi-Directional Charging:

V2G Technology: Advancements in Vehicle-to-Grid (V2G) technology enable electric vehicles to not only receive power from the grid but also contribute stored energy back to the grid, enhancing energy flexibility.

5. Solar-Powered Chargers:

Enhanced Efficiency: Ongoing developments in solar charging technology aim to improve efficiency and reliability, making solar-powered chargers more practical and efficient for various devices.

6. Adaptive Charging Algorithms:

AI-Powered Charging: Integration of artificial intelligence (AI) in charging systems enables adaptive and optimized charging patterns based on device requirements, usage behavior, and available power sources.

7. Eco-Friendly Charging Solutions:

Renewable Energy Integration: Chargers incorporating renewable energy sources such as solar or wind power contribute to eco-friendly charging solutions, supporting sustainable energy usage.

8. Smart Grid Integration:

Efficient Energy Distribution: Chargers integrated with smart grid technology facilitate optimized energy distribution, reducing wastage and promoting efficient charging practices.

9. Ultra-Fast Charging:

Breakthroughs in Charging Speeds: Ongoing research aims to develop ultra-fast charging solutions that can provide a full charge to devices in a matter of minutes, revolutionizing charging times.

10. Multi-Device Charging Solutions:

Simultaneous Charging: Chargers designed to power multiple devices simultaneously, utilizing advanced circuitry to distribute power efficiently among connected gadgets.

Emerging trends in charger technology reflect a shift towards faster, more efficient, and eco-conscious charging solutions.

These advancements hold promise for revolutionizing how we charge our devices, offering convenience, speed, and sustainability. As innovation continues to drive the field forward, these trends pave the way for a future where charging is not only seamless and swift but also environmentally friendly and adaptable to diverse energy sources.

PREDICTIONS FOR THE FUTURE OF CHARGING DEVICES

The landscape of charging devices is on an evolutionary trajectory, constantly innovating to meet the increasing demands for faster, more efficient, and eco-friendly power solutions. Predicting the future of charging devices involves envisioning advancements driven by technological breakthroughs, consumer needs, and sustainability goals. Here's a glimpse into the potential predictions for the future of charging devices:

1. Ultra-Fast Charging Becomes the Norm:

Anticipate advancements in charging technologies that will significantly reduce charging times. Ultra-fast charging solutions could potentially provide a full charge within a few minutes, revolutionizing the way we power our devices.

2. Universal Standardization with USB-C Power Delivery:

USB-C Power Delivery is likely to become the universal standard for charging across various devices due to its versatility, fast-charging capabilities, and compatibility across a wide range of gadgets.

3. Wireless Charging Revolutionizes Mobility:

Wireless charging innovations will progress to extend beyond smartphones and tablets. Expect advancements in wireless charging technology for larger devices, such as laptops, and even vehicles, facilitating hassle-free and efficient charging on-the-go.

4. Eco-Friendly and Sustainable Charging Solutions Prevail:

The emphasis on sustainability will drive the development of chargers integrated with renewable energy sources like solar or kinetic energy, promoting eco-friendly charging solutions while reducing dependency on traditional power grids.

5. Smart and Adaptive Charging Systems Dominate:

The integration of artificial intelligence (AI) into charging systems will enable smarter, more adaptive charging algorithms. AI-powered chargers will optimize power distribution based on usage patterns, device requirements, and energy availability.

6. Multi-Device Charging Solutions Become Standard:

Chargers capable of simultaneously powering multiple devices will gain prominence. These advanced chargers will efficiently allocate power among various gadgets, catering to the growing demand for multi-device usage.

7. Breakthroughs in Battery Technology:

Anticipate advancements in battery technology, including the adoption of solid-state batteries, lithium-sulfur batteries, or other novel chemistries. These innovations promise higher energy densities, faster charging, and enhanced safety compared to current lithium-ion batteries.

8. Integration of Charging Technology into Everyday Objects:

Expect to see charging technology integrated into everyday objects, such as furniture, surfaces, and wearables, enabling seamless and wireless power transfer without the need for dedicated charging stations.

9. Enhanced Focus on Safety and Standards:

With the proliferation of charging devices, a heightened focus on safety standards, compliance, and regulatory measures will be crucial to ensure user safety and mitigate potential hazards associated with evolving charging technologies.

10. Continued Collaboration and Innovation:

Collaboration between tech companies, researchers, and energy experts will drive continuous innovation, resulting in more efficient, accessible, and sustainable charging solutions that cater to the evolving needs of consumers and industries.

The future of charging devices promises a revolutionary transformation in how we power our gadgets. Anticipate a landscape where speed, efficiency, sustainability, and adaptability converge to offer charging solutions that not only meet but exceed the expectations of consumers while aligning with the global pursuit of a greener and more connected future.

As technology continues to evolve, the realm of charging devices will undoubtedly shape a more efficient, convenient, and eco-friendly world of power solutions.

IMPLICATIONS FOR HEALTH AND WELLNESS

In the era of pervasive technology, the implications of charging devices on health and wellness have garnered attention due to their omnipresence in our daily lives. While charging devices enable connectivity and convenience, considerations regarding their impact on health and well-being are vital. Here's an exploration of the implications associated with charging devices:

1. Electromagnetic Fields (EMFs) and Health:

Exposure Concerns: Charging devices emit low levels of electromagnetic fields (EMFs). While extensive research suggests that typical exposure is safe, prolonged and close-range exposure may raise concerns for some individuals, prompting them to minimize EMF exposure.

2. Blue Light Emission and Sleep Disruption:

Impact on Circadian Rhythms: Screens and charging devices emit blue light, which can interfere with the body's production of melatonin, disrupting sleep patterns. Charging devices used before bedtime may contribute to sleep disturbances.

3. Psychological Impact and Stress:

Digital Dependency: Excessive screen time associated with charging devices, particularly smartphones, can lead to increased stress, anxiety, and psychological strain due to constant connectivity and information overload.

4. Physical Effects and Safety Concerns:

Heat Generation: Charging devices, especially during rapid charging or wireless charging, can generate excess heat, potentially impacting battery longevity and causing discomfort or safety concerns if devices become excessively hot.

5. Sedentary Behavior and Health Risks:

Prolonged Screen Time: Charging devices often promote sedentary behaviors, contributing to a more inactive lifestyle and increasing the risk of health issues such as obesity, cardiovascular problems, and musculoskeletal disorders.

6. Digital Addiction and Mental Well-being:

Dependency and Disconnect: Excessive use of charging devices may lead to digital addiction, affecting mental health, social interactions, and overall well-being by creating a disconnect from the real world.

7. Impact on Children and Development:

Behavioral and Cognitive Development: Children's exposure to charging devices, if not moderated, may affect cognitive development, attention span, and social skills, raising concerns about the long-term impact on their well-being.

8. Striking a Balance:

Mindful Usage: Promoting mindful and moderate usage of charging devices, taking breaks, and establishing boundaries can mitigate potential health implications and foster a more balanced relationship with technology.

While charging devices offer unparalleled convenience and connectivity, their implications on health and wellness warrant attention. Achieving a harmonious balance between the benefits of technology and the potential risks requires a mindful approach, incorporating moderation, setting boundaries, and fostering awareness to mitigate adverse effects on physical, mental, and emotional well-being. Understanding the implications of charging devices on health is crucial in navigating a digitally connected world while prioritizing holistic well-being.

CHAPTER 12: EMPOWERING A CHARGED-UP FUTURE

TIPS FOR RESPONSIBLE CHARGER USAGE

Responsible charger usage is essential for ensuring the safety of devices, conserving energy, and minimizing potential risks associated with charging devices. Adopting mindful practices and implementing safety measures can contribute to a safer and more sustainable charging experience. Here are some tips for responsible charger usage:

1. Use Certified and Genuine Chargers:

Utilize chargers that are certified by reputable organizations such as CE, UL, or FCC to ensure compliance with safety standards and compatibility with your devices.

2. Avoid Overloading Outlets:

Refrain from plugging multiple chargers into a single outlet to prevent overheating or potential fire hazards. Use power strips or surge protectors if necessary.

3. Inspect Charging Cables Regularly:

Check charging cables for signs of wear, fraying, or exposed wires. Damaged cables should be replaced immediately to prevent electrical hazards.

4. Unplug Chargers When Not in Use:

Disconnect chargers from power outlets when not actively charging devices to avoid unnecessary energy consumption and reduce standby power usage, known as vampire power.

5. Mindful Charging Practices:

Avoid overcharging devices, as continuous charging after reaching 100% can degrade the battery life over time. Unplug devices once they're fully charged.

6. Optimize Charging Times:

Charge devices during off-peak hours to contribute to energy efficiency and reduce strain on the power grid, especially for larger appliances or electric vehicles.

7. Choose Energy-Efficient Chargers:

Opt for energy-efficient chargers that have high-efficiency ratings and comply with energy-saving standards, contributing to reduced power consumption.

8. Charge Devices in Well-Ventilated Areas:

Place charging devices on non-flammable surfaces in well-ventilated areas to prevent overheating and ensure proper air circulation during charging.

9. Educate Children about Charger Safety:

Teach children about the safe use of chargers, emphasizing the importance of handling them responsibly and avoiding mishandling or tampering.

10. Dispose of Old or Damaged Chargers Properly:

Recycle or dispose of old, damaged, or obsolete chargers responsibly at designated e-waste recycling centers to prevent environmental pollution.

11. Avoid Counterfeit Chargers:

Be cautious of purchasing counterfeit or uncertified chargers, as they may pose safety risks and potentially damage devices due to poor quality and lack of safety standards.

12. Consider Energy-Efficient Charging Solutions:

Explore eco-friendly charging options such as solar-powered chargers or energy-efficient adapters to minimize reliance on traditional electricity sources.

Responsible charger usage entails adopting mindful practices to ensure safety, conserve energy, and promote sustainability. By implementing these tips and incorporating responsible charging habits into daily routines, individuals can contribute to a safer and more eco-conscious approach to charging devices while prolonging the lifespan of gadgets and minimizing environmental impact. Prioritizing responsible charger usage is a small yet significant step towards creating a safer and more sustainable technological environment.

PROMOTING A HEALTHY TECH LIFESTYLE

In today's digitally connected world, maintaining a healthy relationship with technology is crucial for overall well-being. A healthy tech lifestyle involves mindful and purposeful engagement with devices while prioritizing physical, mental, and emotional health. Here's a guide on how to promote a healthy tech lifestyle:

1. Set Boundaries and Tech-Free Zones:

Establish Tech-Free Times: Designate specific periods during the day for disconnecting from devices to focus on other activities, fostering a healthy balance.

2. Practice Mindful Technology Use:

Intentional Engagement: Be mindful of the time spent on devices, focusing on productive activities, and avoiding mindless scrolling or excessive screen time.

3. Prioritize Real-Life Connections:

Quality Face-to-Face Interactions: Foster meaningful relationships by prioritizing in-person interactions and quality time with family and friends over virtual communication.

4. Manage Screen Time:

Set Screen Time Limits: Use screen time management tools to monitor and limit daily usage, especially for children, ensuring a balanced approach to device usage.

5. Balance Tech Use with Physical Activity:

Incorporate Exercise: Pair tech use with physical activities or exercise routines to counterbalance sedentary behavior associated with screen time.

6. Practice Digital Detox and Unplug:

Periodic Disconnect: Schedule regular digital detox sessions or tech-free days to unwind, relax, and engage in offline activities for mental rejuvenation.

7. Prioritize Mental Health:

Limit Exposure to Negative Content: Protect mental health by curating positive and meaningful content and reducing exposure to negativity or stress-inducing information online.

8. Foster Awareness and Education:

Tech Literacy: Promote awareness about healthy tech habits among children, adults, and the elderly, emphasizing responsible and balanced tech use.

9. Model Healthy Tech Behaviors:

Lead by Example: Demonstrate healthy tech habits by setting a positive example for others, balancing your tech use, and maintaining a healthy lifestyle.

10. Practice Self-Care and Mindfulness:

Mindful Tech Breaks: Take breaks during tech use to practice mindfulness, relaxation exercises, or breathing techniques to reduce stress and recharge.

11. Disconnect Before Bedtime:

Create a Tech-Free Bedtime Routine: Disconnect from devices at least an hour before bedtime to improve sleep quality and promote better rest.

12. Seek Support and Balance:

Seek Balance: Regularly reassess and adjust tech usage habits to find a balance that aligns with your lifestyle and contributes to overall well-being.

Promoting a healthy tech lifestyle involves conscious and intentional use of technology to support well-being, balance, and fulfillment. By adopting mindful practices, setting boundaries, and prioritizing real-life connections and self-care, individuals can cultivate a healthier relationship with technology, fostering a more balanced and fulfilling life in the digital age. Striking a harmonious balance between technology and well-being is essential for navigating the digital world while prioritizing mental, physical, and emotional health.

CONCLUSION

In the illuminating journey through "Voltage Health: Exploring the Link Between Chargers and Wellness," author Sam Swinton intricately navigates the intricate relationship between our charging devices and our overall well-being. The book delves into the often-overlooked nexus between technology and health, offering insightful perspectives, practical guidance, and thought-provoking considerations.

Throughout the pages of this comprehensive exploration, Swinton artfully addresses the multifaceted impact of charging devices on our physical, mental, and emotional health. From examining the implications of electromagnetic fields (EMFs) to elucidating responsible charging practices and fostering a balanced tech lifestyle, the book serves as a compass in navigating the complexities of our digital age.

By elucidating the implications, challenges, and opportunities presented by our interactions with chargers and technology, Swinton underscores the importance of mindfulness, education, and responsible usage. The book empowers readers with knowledge, encouraging a more conscious and intentional approach to tech engagement while promoting the prioritization of well-being.

"Voltage Health" not only raises pertinent questions but also provides actionable insights, enabling readers to make informed choices and strike a harmonious balance between the conveniences of technology and the preservation of personal wellness. Sam Swinton's meticulous research, practical advice, and emphasis on sustainable, safe, and mindful tech habits resonate deeply, emphasizing the significance of a healthy relationship with our devices.

As we conclude this insightful journey, "Voltage Health" leaves us with a poignant reminder: the fusion of technology and well-being necessitates a conscious, balanced approach.

With this newfound understanding, readers are poised to embark on a path toward a more harmonious coexistence with technology—a path that prioritizes wellness, embraces responsible practices, and fosters a healthier, more fulfilling digital life.

"Voltage Health" stands not just as a testament to the intricate link between chargers and wellness but as a guidepost, urging us to tread thoughtfully in the realm where technology and well-being intersect—a realm where informed choices pave the way toward a healthier, more balanced tomorrow.